The Regimen

Grow Your Natural Hair Fast

Chapters

Chapter 1: The Introduction

Is your hair hard to manage? Does it break off every time you comb or brush it? What am I doing wrong...you may wonder? Why Isn't my hair growing. Maybe you have a relaxer in and are dreading the "big chop". Maybe you have been natural for an amount of time and just cant seem to get your hair to grow. The question is not what your doing wrong. It's what your not doing at all!

My goal is to create an exciting book that includes a regimen that you can use to grow out your beautiful black hair to its greatest lengths. Regardless if your natural, relaxed, or in between. Regardless of where your at in your hair journey, you can overcome the natural hair battle. With the proper care you can get optimal results that will give you the most desirable and coveted hair that women everywhere seek.

I will show you with a little time, proper methods, and a little prayer....your hair will grow long and beautiful just like the celebrities you see on television. It doesn't take much. A little water, a little conditioner, and a little time to get the beautiful hair that you've always wanted.

Chapter 1: Since the Beginning

If your like me ever since you were a little girl playing with Barbie, you wanted long beautiful hair. But the truth is, for most black girls, nine times out of ten your mother through a relaxer in your hair before you even got your first menstrual period. From there the long hair battle was down hill.

We all struggle with the "Becky" syndrome. If it's not Becky that you want your hair to be like, then its probably the Kardashian chics that your striving to resemble thru makeup hair and style. But let's face it, long hair is and always has been a hard to reach goal for most!

Let's keep it real! We have a lot of work to do. So before you get started, reading about how to achieve long natural hair... let me take you back a little to how I became a naturalista. Let me share with you how I became knowledgeable about natural hair. You will see that through my education and experience, I have learned the science of black hair care.

Yes ladies I have been to cosmetology school and currently hold an Esthetician License in Florida. If you didn't know, estheticians are trained to treat hair and scalps. No, we're not just doing facials all day. We also do hair treatments too!

Chapter 2: The Beginning

I was wearing my hair natural and decided to relax it again in February of 2014. Since I had gone to hair school in 2008 and obtained 500 hours towards a natural hair license in Huntsville, Alabama. I was fond of relaxing my hair myself. Besides many stylist have a bad reputation of cutting too much off the ends, or over relaxing. Honestly, I hate salons. I only go....well I don't go! Ever.

However, in the middle of my relaxed shoulder length hair I decided because I had 2 jobs and was making a little money, I would treat myself to a hair stylist.

Big mistake!

Why did i ever do that. I met a stylist from craigslist who claimed to do $35 blow outs to perfection. She called herself doing... a "silk press", which wasn't silky when she finished. It was cute because she flipped the ends like Nia Long's famous short hair style. But for a shoulder length head of hair....I expected more "oomph". So I paid my $35 and even gave her a $15 tip toward the next style. I walked out the salon happy that day. Feeling that I was on my way to beautiful long natural hair. Boy did I make a mistake.

Later, after the hair style that only lasted a week had worn off, I decided to glue and put some weave in my hair. Instead of paying for a sew-in, I decided to glue in some hair on my own. After all how much damage could it do? No big deal right? Wrong......I am still crying about that decision to this day.

Its not that I had put the glue in (Bad choice but not fatal) but the fact that I decided to go back to the same stylist and let her take the weave and glue out relying on her expertise. What a fool I was. In previous years, I had discovered a shampoo and conditioner from Sally's (The orange and white bottle by ION) that dissolves hair glue without an issue....so why I didn't use it this day. Sure beats me.

So there I was...in the shampoo chair at my stylist as she tugged away at the glue and my beautiful shoulder length hair. I could actually hear and feel my hair rip out as she yanked at my head. I wanted to cry! But how bad could it be. I mean what relaxed *diva* hasn't experienced some breakage with the glue in method. Its normal I thought. It couldn't be that bad right?

I was so wrong. When I got up out the chair, chunks of my hair were missing in the middle, the top, and only God knows where else. I wanted to scream "GOD HELP ME" but I just took it as a lost. I thought to myself … Never again. I paid her and left angry!

I have not been back to a stylist since and after trying to re-cooperate from the damage by getting kinky twist. I realized the unthinkable. It was time for the *BIG CHOP*. In may of 2015 I cut most of my hair off to start over.

After the big chop I went in like crazy with dish washing liquid and vinegar to strip and remove my perm. (YES ITS CRAZY BUT IT WORKS). I had about 1 inch of hair left and with tears in my eyes. I began the transition. From relaxed to natural. It's 2016 now and my hair is beautiful, natural and curly. Not to mention it is growing longer every day. I make my own products most of the time and I am on a mission to grow long and beautiful hair down to my ankles. I will have bra strap length hair and the most beautiful 4c texture and shine ever for certain.

I don't measure my hair much but the last time I measured my hair I was like wow. I discovered that my hair grows an average of ½ to 1 inch every two weeks to a month. I know that I am doing the right thing for my hair. People ask me questions about my natural hair all the time. This is why I'm sharing my secret with you that I have learned from women with long beautiful hair! Although you can find most of this information online, I believe that it is helpful to keep a manual handy to hold yourself accountable to the techniques and routines that I teach you in this book. So please, read on..... enjoy yourself!

Chapter 3: The science of Hair

Have you ever been told that black hair is different from white hair? Well it's a lie, to an extent!

It's a little white lie, until you start to realize a few things. Hair is hair. What makes hair grow is proper care. What makes hair fall out is rough, lack of maintenance and care. Over processing, over heating, and over stressing hair will make it dry, split, and eventually break off. That's not what you want! The genetic makeup of African American hair, is no different than Caucasian hair....other than the curl pattern, there is no difference. Each hair strand is the same. Now if your expecting to hear details about the hair follicle structure and tell you all kind of nonsense about the roots and the structural makeup of hair.... this is not the right book! If you want to learn about hair to that extent I suggest you buy a cosmetology book by Milady's. This is the book they use in beauty school to teach about hair.

However, what I am presenting to you is the truth, minus all the scientific facts. Besides, all you really want is longer hair right! If I spent my time writing about the hair and it's structural makeup you would be bored to death. Now I'm not saying that hair school is not exciting... I'm just saying that I prefer to just get right to the point..... so you can learn what works without wasting time.

So let's keep it simple. Black hair is course, comes in different textures. Some may have a 4c pattern, others may have the toughest to deal with 4b textures like myself. There are a lot of post and websites about the different types of hair out there, this is not it.

In addition, black hair is general dry and brittle compared to our European counterparts. Their hair is silky straight and appears to be longer. You may have even heard that you cannot wash your hair every day. For the most part this is not true. It's only true when you discuss the fact that the natural oils will be stripped by the shampoo in daily washing. But I'm here to tell you there is a way that you can wash your hair every day. While I only wash my hair once a month. I co-wash my hair twice a week. Once on Monday and again on Friday. If your not sure what co-washing please continue reading. The next chapter will discuss products.

From this day forward, the only thing that you need to know about the science of hair is that cosmetology school teaches students that all hair is alike. So whether your Korean or Spanish, African American or European Your hair genetic makeup is the same. We all have a scalp, roots and ends that are made up of the basics which include a sebaceous gland, hair bulb, papilla, sheath, cuticle, and cortex.

What they all mean to you is irrelevant, because regardless of how curly or fine your hair is.....you only have to do a few simple things to get it to grow. These steps include co wash-n- detangle, rinse and balance your ph, condition and oil, moisture and seal the strands, and finally choose between protective styling and minimize heat. Yes ladies, it's that simple. Continue to read and you will see!

Chapter 4: Definitions and Terms

This chapter is plain and easy to understand. There is no point in learning a lesson bout your sebaceous glands, hair bulb, papilla, sheath, cuticle, and cortex unless your going to become a hair stylist. I am not qualified to teach you those things so I will not even attempt to do so. You don't have to worry about it. For the sake of this chapter. You need to know a few basic terms. These terms are easy to understand.

The first definition is **co-washing**, which in my regimen you will see allows you to completely forget about shampooing your hair because it results in drying out the hair. Most shampoos are harsh and strip the natural hair oils simply use the method. Co-washing is the method of substituting shampoo for conditioner easy and plain. You simply follow the instructions on the conditioner or co-wash product and move on to the next step. Because of the recent request and buzz about co-washing some brands like As I Am are resulting to creating co-washing products which include only a small amount of shampoo ingredient mixed with more of a conditioning agent.

The next term is **finger detangling.** Finger detangling takes the place of brushing or combing. In this simple hair regimen you can throw out your hair brush and comb if you'd like because it is simply not needed to grow long hair. In fact there is even a young lady on YouTube who has booty-length hair that hasn't brushed or combed her hair in years. If you would like to keep your comb that is fine however you need to know to get your hair to grow the lack of manipulation is important. Combs have been known to break the hair and cause damage. So choose wisely.

Next you need to know about **manipulation.** Manipulation is can be defined as anything that touches the hair, such as brushing, combing, styling and so forth. For the sake of your hair, manipulation is detrimental to it's growth. You have always heard the term less is more, well it is true. The less you mess with your hair, the more it will grow.

Detangling your hair is a well known term. Detangling refers to the process of getting rid of knots and tangles in the hair. As until recent, a comb has been used to detangle but I am encouraging you to throw out your comb and stare to finger detangle your hair. **Finger Detangling** is when you use your fingers and hands to get out the knots. This process is a little bit more tedious and requires a little more time for longer hair, but will eventually be easy once you get your hair regimen going.

Rinse or Rinsing your hair is easy. The it is the method of washing out your products which at most for the sake of this hair care regimen will only include co-wash conditioners, oils, moisturizers or deep conditioners. You will also learn about **Balancing your ph**. After you wash your hair with co-wash and finger detangle you need to balance your hair ph with a natural ph balancing solution. You will later learn about the use of apple cider vinegar as a ph balancing agent to help your hair stay soft and manageable.

Conditioner or Deep conditioner is also a term you need to know if you don't already. This is the process of applying a product to leave in the hair for 5 minutes or more to help the hair absorb moisture and nutrients.

Moisturize or Moisturizing refers to the technique of applying a water based creme or solution such as a leave-in-conditioner to the hair to keep the hair strands moist. This step should be followed by a hair oil to seal the strands.

How to Oil your hair is also discussed in this regimen, but for now you need to know the definition of **Oil**. Please be aware that for this hair care regimen just any ole oil will not work. Although there are plenty of popular brands of hair oil, you should rely on the more natural products that won't dry the hair out. Most oils on the market are mixed with other products such as glycerin or alcohols. Just remember after you moisturize your hair you will need to seal your strands with oil to keep the moisture locked in.

Heat Protection refers to the popular products and process of using a heat minimizing agent on the hair before you blow dry or press the hair with a flat iron. Until now pressing oils and greases have been very popular but despite popular demand the African American community has been left with short dry and breaking brittle hair. With the lack of a proper heat protection your hair is going to fry under the flat iron during the heating process. A simple hair grease will not do!

Protective Styles are when you use hair braiding, twisting, dreading, buns and covering to keep your hair ends out of the way. Although some would disagree, if your not using tight hair bands or rubber to restrict your hair a simple bun or ponytail can be considered a protective style also.

Chapter 5: Products and Care

Products and Care is a touchy subject in any hair community. So I while I cannot tell you what products to use or not, I can give you an Idea of some products that I have used in the past prior to starting my own natural hair growth rapidly.

Some of my previous favorite products are Doo Gro Stimulating growth oil. I used this product every day for years when I was younger. I used to press my hair on the stove with a comb. I used to leave a section of my hair out in the front to cover the tracks when I got a sew in. I would use the Doo Gro as a heat protection against the 450+ degree heat to keep the left out section of my hair from breaking. To my surprise my hair would never break in the front. This stuff is strong and structurally sound. It's also good to oil the scalp and helps your hair grow at its maximum rate. If you haven't tried it you should.

Next on my list of products is Cantu, however until recently they have not had natural hair lines for blacks. Anyhow their products are awesome and very good to maintain the hair. I don't like all of their products but they at least deserve a mention. Feel free to implement their products in to this regimen.

SheaMoisture is a great product as well. Although I have no favorite from their line, I have used it in the past to help me get my hair to where it is today. They have great deep conditioners that the online hair community is crazy about. I feel they are worth a try.

Next up excitingly is a new product I discovered called Shima Hair Oil. The product is developed by a lady named Shima and can be found online at shimahaircare.com She also provides shampoos, leave-in-conditioners, and Shea butters that can help you on your hair journey. The exciting thing about Shima's hair products is that she uses them herself and will write you back if you message her on Facebook. She also does tutorials on YouTube that explain why she has booty-length relaxed African American hair. Her hair is long and beautiful. I encourage you to check her out.

And finally, is my personal growth products. It's right that I would include my own product tips for you. My products are all hand made in the USA and include the bare minimal ingredients with no substitutes. There are no alcohols, no glycerin, and no gunk at all. They are made with natural and organic ingredients to help you are for your beautiful natural or relaxed hair. The product line is formulated for all hair types, but is great for hair that needs moisture. The final chapter will be about my hair products. I will tell you how to order them although it is not required of you, I believe they can help you achieve the long hair that you desire.

Chapter 6: The Regimen Overview

If you've made it this far you are probably saying that I can do this! Yes you can. You have made it to the 6th chapter, and if you stop reading here you will know everything you need to know about my regimen in an over view. Although I suggest you read the whole book, this chapter alone is very conclusive to get you started.

<u>The Regimen</u>

1. Wash your hair using a conditioner or co-wash product. Using Luke Warm Water. Get rid of your Shampoo you will never need it again.
2. Finger Detangling. Throw out your combs and brushes. Use your fingers.
3. Rinse Using an Apple Cider Vinegar, or **a good Ph Rinse Like Alphogee PH 2 Step Treatment**
4. Deep condition hair for 30 minutes under a plastic cap. Use Body Heat!
5. Rinse again using cool water only. Follow by a finger detangle again.
6. Moisturize the hair with a leave in conditioner or moisturizer.

7. Apply hair Oil from ends to roots. Do not get on scalp. Dry your hair.

8. Use heat protection if you must flat iron or curl your hair.

9. Chose a Protective Style or Leave the hair down.

10. Apply water, moisturizers, and oils through the day to keep the hair in a soft manageable condition.

Chapter 7: Co-washing your hair

As you may have learned by now. I barely use shampoo to wash my hair. I may use shampoo once a month, but only if it's a natural product. Even then it's only if my scalp needs a Deep serious cleanse. Other than that I co-wash.

Co-washing is great for all hair. There is no reason that you can't achieve the look and length that you desire by using a conditioner or co-washing product for your hair regimen. Shampoo is a thing of the past!

To co-wash your hair, if your hair is long may take a longer amount of time than if it was short. However the process is very similar for both. If your hair is long wet it til damp with warm water. Using warm water opens the hair follicles and gets therm ready to receive the product. If your hair is short simply wetting it with warm water will do.

Next you need to apply the co-wash/conditioner to your hair from ends to root. If your hair is long you can do this in sections. Some people say that you don't have to wash your roots, however I disagree. It will not hurt you to get the product on your scalp. It's made for hair. After all up until now you've been washing your hair with shampoo and it hasn't done any harm. Conditioners and Co-washes are much milder than shampoos and do not strip the hair of their natural moisture. And finally rinse the hair using mild warm or cold water.

Chapter 8: Finger Detangling

After you co-wash your hair, you need to finger detangle it. If your hair is in sections, detangle each section individually. However, for shorter hair, simply use your hands to gently detangle and get rid of hair knots. Detangling the hair can be frustrating.

However if you co-wash your hair and rinse it all in one direction it will become easier over time.

To correctly detangle the hair, detangle it from ends to root. Be sure to not apply excessive force or stretch the hair too much. It will break off if you are not careful. Although there may be sections of your hair that require a comb, try to avoid it as much as possible.

Apply conditioner if you need help detangling the hair. The conditioner can help the hair obtain more slip and detangle easier. Be sure that you don't detangle from root to ends. This is not the way to treat your hair if you want it to grow. It may cause the hair to weaken or come out at the roots.

Be gentle with your hair. The detangle process is the hardest part of my hair regimen so take your time. If you are in a rush to detangle, don't do it.

Place a cap or a wig on until you have time to actually go through the hair little by little. For shorter hair, detangling can be easier. Remember less manipulation is best!

Chapter 9: The Rinse Method

The rinse method is not as hard as it sounds. Up until now you may or may not have a lot of product in your hair and you have already finger detangled it. You are over the hard part, detangling.

Rinsing your hair is easy or so it seams but if you don't do it right with the correct technique you can do more damage to your hair than you think. Are you rinsing your hair under a sing? Are you laying in the tub? Is your hair down or up? How many times are you rinsing your hair? All of the answers to these questions matter.

If your rinsing your hair under as ink, be sure to not scratch at or tangle the hair again. Do not do the famous "stylist" method where they mix all the hair together trying to get the product out. Rinse the hair in one easy direction, slow and easy. This will help you minimize additional tangling. Besides having to detangle your hair too many times is annoying and time consuming.

If your rinsing in the tub laying down or in the shower stand up, the same applies. Rinse the hair in one easy motion. Place your head backwards under the water to ensure that all the water gets out. Rinsing in the tub can be a good or bad thing depending on if the water is already dirty or not. However it is a great way to minimize detangling and additional breakage.

Rinse with cool water to close the hair follicles, and be sure to detangle.

Chapter 10: Balancing your Ph

After you finally have your hair rinsed and detangled. You may or may not have time to balance your ph. The natural ph of hair and scalp is 4.5 to 5.5, and if you didn't know depending on the product you use your ph can be lower or higher than the recommended. This is why you will occasionally need to implement the ph balancing phase to your regimen to keep your hair in check.   Hair/Lower ph than recommended can break or become very dry or damaged. We don't want this! As of now there are not a lot of products on the market good for balancing the ph. Some products like Head and Shoulder claim to balance the ph. However, in my Esthetician school they talked about how horrible the product was. Whether this or true or not, I have a cheap solution that is sure to work. Apple cider vinegar is awesome for your hair. It will balance your ph and leave your hair soft as a baby's butt. I have to give credit to Danielle Matthews for teaching me this technique a few years ago. No wonder hear hair is long and beautiful!

ACV also makes a product consuption easy for balancing your ph. It cost a little bit more than apple cider vinegar but it is worth every dime! Once you apply your apple cider vinegar or **any** Ph balancing solution, rinse the hair out with cool water. Remember keep the hair in one direction to minimize detangling.

When your done balancing your ph, your hair should be ready to receive the best treatment of all. The conditioner. At this point you have already washed your hair with conditioner or a co-washing product. So you may decide to leave this process for those days when your hair needs extra conditioner.

For the most part Deep conditioning can be done once every week, bi-weekly, or once a month. Because all hair types are different some hair may need more deep conditioners than others. I personally deep condition two to three times a week. I often leave the deep conditioner in over night or for hours at a time. My hair is extremely dry and I am still learning how to keep it moisturized

There is no such thing as over conditioning the hair. It will not hurt your hair to deep condition it every day. If white people can do it you can too....because remember the science and genetic makeup of hair is the same. The only time I would make an exception to this rule is when it comes to shampoos that are harsh and dry out the hair's natural oils. Don't even think about it!

When applying deep conditioner apply it from the ends to the roots, try not to get it in the scalp. It may contain oils and other things that you wont want to clog your pores. After you deep condition, rinse the hair and always detangle.

Chapter 12: Moisturize and Seal

Now that your hair has a balanced ph and is conditioned, you need to apply a moisturizer. If you think that oils will work by themselves, they wont.

While oils are great for the hair, they have a consistency that resist water, so you need to apply a moisturizing product.

There are plenty of moisturizers on the market. You can choose a leave-in-conditioner or even a regular conditioner to leave in your hair. However, I can recommend a great product called Africa's Best Hair Mayonnaise. I have been using this hair product for years and it leaves my hair soft and manageable every time!

ACV usage also makes moisturizers for the hair that are natural with no substitutes or junk smoother on application. The products after ACV applied, are great for natural hair or hair that needs extra moisture. Good products should Shea butters, olive oils, and natural solutions for obtaining moisture. Just remember that a good moisturizer usually comes in a creamy solution that is easy to pour or scoop out.

Some people may use Shea butter as a moisturizer, however the whipped Shea butter is the best form to use. Unrefined Shea butters are also great for moisturizing because they absorb the hair. However until the hair absorbs the moisture the hair can be left feeling heave. For the purpose of moisturizing the lighter your hair feels the better.

Chapter 13: How to Oil Your Hair

After you moisturize your hair you need to seal your ends with an oil. Remember not just any oil will do. Honestly if your finding your oil on the shelf at Walmart, you may need to think again. Other than Doo Gro oils, I would not recommend you to seal your hair with an oil from the beauty store.

Remember to seal your hair from ends to root in that order!

Oils such as jojoba, olive or argan are best. Don't be fooled, not all oils are created equal. While I was in Esthetician school I learned some devastating truth! The FDA does not regulate hair products so if a product makes claim that it is natural and it is on the shelf, it may or may not be. You need to really do your research and make sure that the product is natural. I also learned that just because it says natural on the bottle does not mean that the product is 100% natural. Without the regulation of the FDA products lines can use the word "natural' or "organic" to describe one or two ingredients in their product, while the rest of the ingredients are synthetics and they will not get in any trouble. Nobody really knows what products are real or not anymore. This is why I created my own products. I get my ingredients from a well known natural and organic supplier here inside the USA that have all their ingredients approved to be certified organics by the FDA. You can't go wrong with **organic products.**

Chapter 14: Heat Protection

Now that your ends are sealed, you will need to use a heat protectant if you plan to use a flat iron, blow dry or curl your hair. I have not used a blow dryer or curling iron in years. However when I did I used Doo Gro Stimulating growth oil to protect my hair. The product does not claim to be a heat protectant but it does work well for a substitute.

If you are not using heat protectants and still using hair greases you need to reconsider. I know we are creatures of habit but this is probably the reason your hair is not growing or is not as long as you would like. You need to reconsider your techniques and products. The only heat protectant that I know of is one by Tresemme, but a lot of hair products carry them. I cannot personally recommend the heat protectant by Tresemme so I cannot tell you about it's quality. However, I do know Tresemme has good conditioners and hair sprays that I have used in the past.

Whatever product you choose to use, be sure that you are not over processing or heating your hair. If you see smoke turn your unit down. I never use heat on my hair. If you must use heat to style and flat iron your hair be sure to use a heat protectant. Over processed or heated hair can be dry brittle and have split ends. Dry hair and split ends break and that is the opposite of what you are trying to achieve.

Chapter 15: Daily Wear and Care

What is your routine for your daily hair care? How are you wearing your hair on a daily basis? Do you wash-n-go? Do you use excessive banding and bows, clip ins and extensions? If your over doing it you should stop. This hair regimen and for the sake of it all, achieving longer hair is about low maintenance styling mixed with high maintenance care.

If your hair is damaged it could be because up until this pint you have done too much heat styling, excessive combing, or wearing braids and weaves too long or too much. Reconsider your daily styling. Think about how easy it is for white women to get get up and go with only a wash and conditioner. You can do this too!

I know you may be saying I cannot go out like this or that, but let me tell you that natural hair, minimal styling are in and weaves are out the door! Although protective styling is recommended by a lot of women in the beauty world, I do not use protective styling other than a wig or a bonnet.

I cover my hair in a bonnet at night after I apply my daily moisturizer and oils. I do not comb my hair every day, and I don't own a brush...blow dryer....or a curling iron. I have a flat iron that I never use and I have not had my hair braided in years. I simply wash-n-go. Whatever your daily routine is, choose wise and minimize!

Your daily regimen should be easy as Becky's daily regimen. Don't over do it. For starters keep your hair moisturized through out the day. This is especially true if your hair is natural. Use a spray bottle to mist your hair with a spray bottle and apply your moisturizer and seal it with an oil as much as needed during the day. Keep your hair soft and fluffy.

If your hair is so dry during the day that you cannot run your fingers through it comfortably then you have a big problem. Moisturize, Moisturize, Moisturize! Oil is not as important is moisturizing, while oil locks the moisture in, water and leave-in-conditioners are what penetrate the hair making the strand swell and remain healthy throughout the day. Some oils do penetrate the hair but for this regimen oils only go on after the moisturizer.

Choose low maintenance styles to wear during the day that allow you to apply moisturizers as much as needed. Braids and weaves make it hard to get to the hair and while many claim they help the hair grow out.....I myself and friends have found that our hair grows faster when we leave it down in order to moisturize and seal it throughout the day as much as needed.

There is nothing like a beautiful head of hair that can blow freely in the wind. So for whatever your daily routine is remember, keep it simple and keep it moisturized.

Chapter 16: Protective Style or Not

This chapter is titled *Protective Style or Not.* You may or may not choose to use protective styling on your hair. While some may find that protective styles such as braids, weaves or twist may grow their hair longer, others may find that it will break their hair off. You have to do what is right for you.

I love to leave my hair down and it brings me joy to run my hands through my hair daily to moisturize and oil it. I believe my hair is beautiful no matter how popular long silky hair may be, I will never again relax my beautiful springy curls. Words cannot express how beautiful it is to me to see my curls stretch out and spring back into place when I apply my **organic products** products to my hair.

I have learned to love my hair in its natural state. I used to get braids and sew ins, and my hair would grow. Because it was not touched and the ends were able to stay protected in the braids. However when I used to get sew ins my hair was over stressed and never grew. This was because of the lack of access I had to my hair during that time in my life.

If you must wear protective styles, wear styles that allow you to reach your hair and moisturize it during the day. Popular protective styles are braids, Bantu knots, kinky twist, french braids and buns. Some do not consider buns to be protective styles but they are. Anything that allows the hair to stay tucked in or out of the way for low manipulation is a protective style. Whatever style you choose minimize tension and maximize daily moisture.

Chapter 17: The Regimen Review

Wow! You did it, you read The Regimen to it's entirety minus a few pages. How do you feel? Isn't my hair regimen easy! It's simple. Let's review.

1. Wet your hair and wash your hair using a conditioner or co-wash product using luke warm water to open the hair follicle.
2. Finger Detangle your hair with conditioner in it to maximize slip. Throw out your combs and brushes and go slow to prevent breakage.
3. Rinse the hair in one direction using an apple cider vinegar, or **organic products Ph Rinse**
4. Whenever you choose Deep condition hair for 30 minutes or more under a plastic cap. Use your body heat to warm the product to minimize heat damage.
5. Rinse your hair again again using cool water this time. Follow by a finger detange if necessary.
6. Moisturize the hair with a leave in conditioner or moisturizer.

7. Apply hair Oil from ends to roots. Do not get on scalp. Dry your hair.

8. Use heat protection if you must flat iron or curl your hair.

9. Choose a Protective Style or Leave the hair down.

10. Apply daily moisturizers and oils to seal the scalp as much as needed. Your hair can never have enough moisture and nutrients.

Chapter 18: organic products Products

Here you are at the final chapter. I hope you are excited about your new regimen. I pray you are on your way to long beautiful hair and decide to try the regimen for yourself. It is a complete and easy routine to help you achieve hair that grows at its optimal ½ to 1 inch per month with proper care. You can do this!

Lastly, although you may have a bathroom full of products I want to introduce you to something that you may find better. I have created a natural hair product called **organic products.** As I mentioned before the products are natural and organic unlike some products that only contain the one to two natural ingredients and then label them as "natural or organic", my products are hand made to perfection.

I do not utilize sweat shops over seas and the products are made in less than a month before you receive them. This means that you will not receive an old product that has been sitting on the counter at the local hair store for months. It means that you will receive a new fresh product with only the best ingredients that will help you obtain the most natural and beautiful length of hair as fast as possible.

organic products is a beautiful product with the lovely scent of Banana Bread unlike any other product on the market it uses a log of a "crown" so that when you receive your product you know it as soon as you see it. I have been mixing products for years since I graduated Florida College of Natural Health in 2011.

I used my knowledge of product ingredients to mix and master the correct volume of Shea butters, olive oils and even aloe Vera gels to give you the maximum results to retain moisture. Did you know your hair may actually be growing at its normal rate. But because you may have split ends or be applying too much heat the ends may be breaking off causing you to think that it is not growing. **organic products** is the perfect product to help you retain those hair ends and keep them sealed. It is my hope that you will consider something new in your hair care regimen. Try **organic products** today!

Well ladies, it's about time that I conclude The Regimen. I hope that you are ready to try something new and get that hair growing! Don't be scared to throw out your hair brush, your comb, and all those nasty products and start a new journey! You deserve it.

Other Facts

Your hair grows ½ an inch per month.

My sometimes grows 1 inch a month with my regime and

products

Protective styles are not necessary

Give your hair a break between protective styles

The FDA does not regulate hair or beauty products

Your favorite natural hair product may not really be natural

Your hair doesn't have to be relaxed to be manageable

Natural hair isn't a trend its a lifestyle

You do not have to trim your hair every 6 to 8 weeks

You should trim your hair only when it needs it

You don't have to trim all your hair at once

You should only trim the hair that needs it

Split ends can ruin your whole head

I only trim my hair every 6 months

You do not have to relax your hair every 6 to 8 weeks

Learning to care for your hair is a long term investment

Natural Hair cost more to maintain than Relaxed hair

Natural hair is not hard to maintain

African American women can grow long beautiful hair

Drinking water helps your hair grow long and beautiful

Eating proper nutrition is important to make your hair grow

longer

For more information on My Books

email me at eliciaonline@gmail.com

To purchase **organic products** products visit

www.bulkapothecary.com :) thats my biggest secret!

Follow organic products:

www.twitter.com/easyesthetics

www.facebook.com/estheticianforlife

www.instagram.com/easyesthetics

visit our blog at

www.easyesthetics.blogspot.com

Thank you for reading The Regimen!

www.easyesthetics.com

www.ingramcontent.com/pod-product-compliance
Lightning Source LLC
Chambersburg PA
CBHW050520290526
45786CB00007B/2627